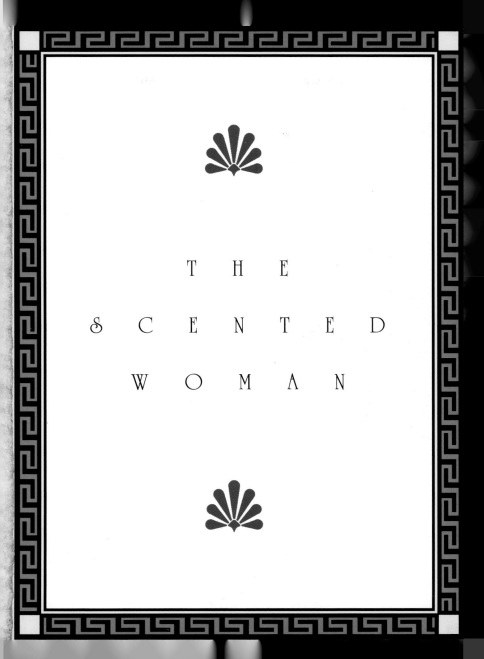

THE SCENTED WOMAN

THE SCENTED WOMAN

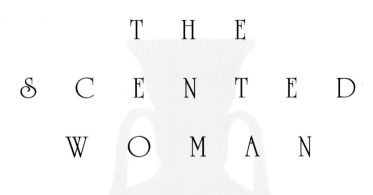

CREATE YOUR OWN SIGNATURE PERFUME

CUSTOM FRAGRANCES BY MARIBETH RIGGS

PAINTINGS BY PABLO PICASSO

VIKING
STUDIO
BOOKS

Note: This book contains recipes using essential oils and other ingredients that, when mixed properly and used externaly, are perfectly safe. However, certain of the contents may cause an allergic reaction in some individuals, so reasonable care in the preparation and use of these perfumes is advised.

VIKING STUDIO BOOKS

Published by the Penguin Group
Viking Penguin, a division of Penguin Books USA Inc., 375 Hudson Street,
New York, New York 10014, U.S.A.
Penguin Books Ltd, 27 Wrights Lane, London W8 5TZ, England
Penguin Books Australia Ltd, Ringwood, Victoria, Australia
Penguin Books Canada Ltd, 10 Alcorn Avenue, Suite 300, Toronto, Ontario, Canada M4V 3B2
Penguin Books (N.Z.) Ltd, 182–190 Wairau Road, Auckland 10, New Zealand

Penguin Books Ltd, Registered Offices: Harmondsworth, Middlesex, England

First published in 1992 by Viking Penguin, a division of Penguin Books USA Inc.

1   3   5   7   9   10   8   6   4   2

LIBRARY OF CONGRESS CATALOGING IN PUBLICATION DATA
Riggs, Maribeth.
The scented woman : create your own signature perfume / custom fragrances
by Maribeth Riggs : paintings by Pablo Picasso.
p.   cm.
Includes bibliographical references.
ISBN 0-670-84117-X
1. Perfumes. 2. Picasso, Pablo, 1881–1973. II. Title.
TP983.R47 1992
668'.54—dc20   91–23708

Printed in Japan

F ⚘ Y
PRODUCTIONS

After bells had rung
 And were silent...
 Flowers chimed
A peal of fragrance

What bloom on what tree
 Yields
 This imperceptible
Essence of incense?

— Basho

Contents

~ 11 ~

Introduction to the Fine Art of Perfumery

~ 17 ~

Delight

A delectable scent that releases slowly and deliciously: fruity Cassis, spicy Vetiver, woody Pine Balsam, and a sweet note of Cinnamon. Redolent of summer, irresistible and joyful.

~ 21 ~

Intrigue

A potent and uninhibited orchestration of rare aromas: Musk, Ambergris, a whisper of Frankincense, and a penetrating top note of Jasmine. A perfume that weaves an intoxicating spell over all who come near.

~ 25 ~

Fresh

A youthful and light composition that enchants every day, anywhere. Top notes of sunny Lemongrass, sweet Orange Blossom, and heavenly Rose are held aloft by the green and woody scents of Rosemary and Sandalwood.

～ 29 ～
TROPICAL

Prepare for a heady jungle-flower adventure. The compelling scents of Gardenia, Ylang-Ylang, Frangipani, and a burst of sweet Cassis float above the earthy Patchouli and Cedarwood base.

～ 33 ～
SPICE

The romance of the Orient captured in a fragrance: East Indian Sandalwood, West Indian Bergamot, Patchouli from Southeast Asia, made piquant with Carnation. A scent for the adventurous.

～ 37 ～
ELEGANT

A worldly perfume with a hypnotic attraction. The subtle essence of Oakmoss is combined with fragrant Bergamot and ethereal Amber to create a scent that lingers in the mind long after it is gone.

～ 41 ～
SERENE

A symphony of intoxicating Rose — the fragrance celebrated by the Sufi poets of Persia — orchestrated with Musk and a lilting note of Sandalwood. An intricate and elevating enchantment.

INNOCENT

A tender flower poem, this disarming concoction is destined to enchant far and wide. Celebrate a Victorian bouquet of timeless floral notes: Lilac, Heliotrope, and Violet. Deliciously subtle, utterly beguiling.

NIGHT

This penetrating, special-occasion scent features Jasmine, the precious flower that exudes its most intense perfume just before dawn. The alluring bouquet is rounded with Amber and Vanilla, and underscored by a woody note of Patchouli. Unforgettable.

SPRING

An outdoor note of Lavender is combined with the clean scent of Rosemary and topped with the gloriously fragrant Tuberose. Bright and fresh, invigorating and inviting.

ESSENTIAL OILS SHOPPING GUIDE

INTRODUCTION TO THE FINE ART OF PERFUMERY

The human fascination with scent is ancient and enduring. Perhaps the earliest use of fragrant plant essences was incense burned as a sacrifice to the gods and goddesses of Mesopotamia. The beautiful, smoky aromas of tree resins — including frankincense, cedar of Lebanon, and myrrh — filled ancient households and sacred temples to attract divine attention.

During the golden age in Egypt, the human body was routinely anointed with all manner of perfumed oils. At first, these "magical" oils were used to increase the personal power of the wearer and to ward off negative influences. As this practice developed, the medicinal and cosmetic uses of aromatic oils became increasingly important. Egyptian priests and scholars invented and perfected a method for extracting plant oil known as enfleurage — a technique that is still in use in the perfume industry today.

Although the Middle East, China, India, and Japan have contributed much to the history of perfumes, Europe eventually became the home of the great perfume manufacturers. The Renaissance exploded with technical advances in the use of aromatic oils for medicine and perfumery. Distillation of pure alcohol provided the first perfume diluent, a neutral substance that prevented the volatile oils from spoiling. With the perfection of glassmaking techniques, plant oils and alcohol could be distilled for the first time with ease and efficiency, and the mass production of perfume began.

Due to the wide variety of fragrances, early perfumers used a form of musical notation to describe scents and simplify the composing of perfume blends. Modern perfume manufacturers have organized these perfume notes into fragrance families. There are six major fragrance families, although new ones are continually developing as synthetic oils are introduced. These six families are floral, green, citrus, Oriental, chypre, and leather/animal. All of these families have smaller divisions within them, and many are combined to achieve certain effects, such as leather/chypre or green/floral. *The Scented Woman* introduces ten original perfumes, all made by combining major and minor perfume notes from the classic perfume families.

The incredible variety of perfume oils that are widely available today presents the opportunity to design a "signature fragrance" to suit any occasion or individual taste. As most perfume wearers know, certain scents induce particular moods or sensations, and they can become an extension of the personality — hence, they become a signature perfume.

The formulas in *The Scented Woman* will allow you to experiment with creating a perfume that may become your own signature scent. To create fragrances in your home, you will need a perfumer's funnel, a glass dropper, several quarter-ounce and one-ounce bottles, diluent, and the essential oils you will be using. Before you begin mixing, lay plastic wrap over your work surface, since essential oils can soak into tabletops and leave behind an indelible odor. Keep paper towels or paper napkins at hand to use as a blotting pad. You'll want to pour diluent in a small, open glass container and keep it nearby as you work, to cleanse the dropper between oils.

Since perfumes can spoil if their containers are not perfectly clean, make sure the bottles you are using are clean and free of dust or dirt particles. Soak the bottles in soapy water and rinse them thoroughly in very hot water before using. Use cotton swabs to dry them thoroughly and allow them to stand upside down overnight before you begin. The containers must be completely dry when you mix the perfume.

All of the formulas in this book require you to mix the perfumes in plain quarter-ounce or one-ounce bottles. Eight formulas will yield perfume-strength compositions and are prepared in quarter-ounce bottles. Two — FRESH and SPRING — are mixed as toilet waters and require one-ounce bottles to accommodate their greater volume. The fragrance formulas call for essential oils, measured in drops, to which you add the diluent. Diluents are commercial formulations that contain unscented alcohol and glycerin, which help combine the oils and preserve the final perfume. If your completed perfume is cloudy, blend in more diluent, five drops at a time, until the oils disperse and the mixture is clear.

Once you have mixed a fragrance, you may use your perfumer's funnel to transfer the blend to a more decorative flask. Again, be certain the flask is perfectly clean. Each of the formulas can also be composed as a bath oil by mixing the blended essential oils with one pint of almond oil in place of the diluent. Or, any formula may be composed as a toilet water by mixing it in a one-ounce bottle.

Most perfumes must age for a few days after they are mixed for their bouquets to fully develop. All perfumes are more stable if they are protected from direct light. Fragrances may be decanted into colored bottles, stored in a medicine cabinet or vanity drawer, or the bottle may be slipped into a velvet pouch. Be sure to store bath oils and bottles of unused essential oils away from the light, as well.

Perfumes and toilet waters can be applied in many ways to experience their maximum effect. Perfume should be applied over major pulse points where the skin is especially warm, which allows the fragrance to "lift" as heat from the body is released. These points are behind the ears, on the wrists, on the inside of the elbows, and on the back of the knees. Perfume can also be applied to the cleavage, to the hollow of the throat, and to the temples. If you are applying toilet water, an atomizer is ideal: spray the fragrance into the air and walk into it, or lightly spray it directly onto the throat, shoulders, wrists, and hair. You may also layer fragrances by bathing in your favorite blend of bath oil and later applying the same blend of perfume or splash of toilet water.

Fine perfumes release their scent over a period of several hours. The first scent to lift from the skin is known as the top note; generally, top notes are the floral essences in the blend. The middle note reflects the perfumer's skill at combining spicy, herbal, woody, or minty essences with higher floral notes. The base note, also known as the dry-out note, is composed of the essential oil fixative that is used to stabilize the blend — most often patchouli, musk, or sandalwood. For a perfume to be a success, all of these notes must unfold pleasantly and harmoniously. Your finished creation will align itself to your specific body chemistry and "lift" exquisitely over a period of several hours.

Beyond the use of perfume as a personal adornment, the fragrance industry is expanding into many other facets of life. The production of "strategic aromas," "productivity perfumes," and "functional fragrances" for use in factories, offices, shopping environments, and even public transportation systems is in development today. Through "olfactory engineering," the scents of the future will be precisely calculated to stimulate physiological responses. On the drawing board are synthetic pheromones and an entire palette of new fragrances on the threshold of commercial use.

For the present, however, you may choose from a large and varied selection of essential oils and perfumer's equipment to engineer your own strategic fragrance. It is very important that you purchase the best-quality essential oils you can find. Good oils can be expensive, but in time you will learn to recognize and appreciate those with rounded, harmonious bouquets. The Essential Oils Shopping Guide at the back of this book lists a number of outlets that carry the oils and perfumer's supplies you will need to get started.

As you learn to identify the scents of the many oils you will be using, you may wish to alter some of the formulas or even create your own compositions. Pages are set aside at the back of the book for you to name and record your new fragrance formulas. If you've never mixed your own perfume, you are in for a fulfilling and often thrilling olfactory adventure.

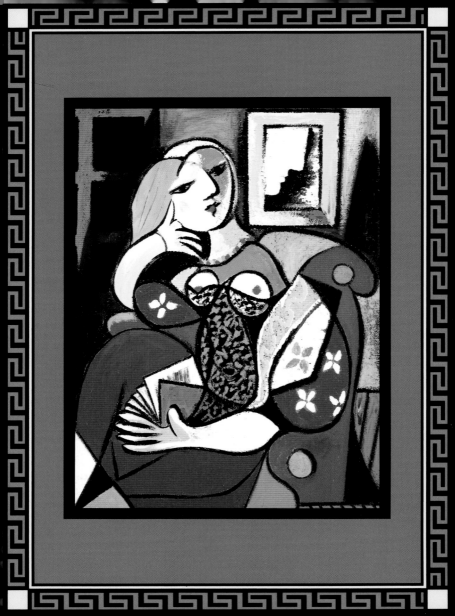

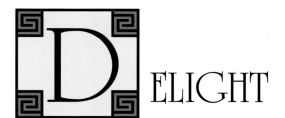

DELIGHT

A delectable scent that

releases slowly and

deliciously: fruity Cassis,

spicy Vetiver,

woody Pine Balsam, and

a sweet note of Cinnamon.

Redolent of summer,

irresistible and joyful.

17

D ELIGHT is a fun-to-wear ambrosia of fruit and spice essences. The base of this festive scent is pine balsam, a contrast note that adds a long-lasting brilliance to the composition.

The spicy, fruitlike cachet of DELIGHT is reminiscent of the famous scent Shéhérazade, designed by Guy Laroche in the 1960s. Laroche brought bold colors and patterns to the world of fashion, and redefined all that was youthful and contemporary. His beautiful Shéhérazade was a captivating blend of cassis and mango, layered with sandalwood and spiced cleverly with nutmeg.

> *60 Drops of Oil of Cassis*
> *9 Drops of Oil of Vetiver*
> *6 Drops of Oil of Cinnamon*
> *6 Drops of Oil of Pine Balsam*
> *Diluent to Fill a Quarter-Ounce Bottle*

A sense of fun and frolic is essential when you select a bottle for DELIGHT. Give in to the offbeat: choose a bottle that is unique and whimsical. Perhaps you will find one in a shape or color that amuses you and reminds you of younger, more carefree days. DELIGHT is formulated as a perfume and will yield one-quarter of an ounce.

Into a quarter-ounce bottle, drop the Oil of Cassis, Oil of Vetiver, Oil of Cinnamon, and Oil of Pine Balsam. Pour or drop in the diluent, filling the bottle almost to the top. Seal the bottle and agitate it lightly to mix; transfer the mixture to your selected scent bottle with a perfumer's funnel. DELIGHT can be worn immediately, and exudes a sweet, uplifting fragrance throughout the day — sure to pique the interest of all who share it.

Cassis, although it is categorized as a floral, is actually a fruit extract taken from the flower bud of the black currant. Usually combined with other floral mixes in small doses, the use of cassis as a body note gives DELIGHT its fruitlike aroma.

Vetiver is classified as a woody minor note on the perfumer's scale. When used in proper proportion, it brings out the best qualities of the fragrances it is blended with. Vetiver is a favorite fixative for light, floral colognes and, as such, anchors the composition with its herbal, peppery flavor.

The bark oil of the cinnamon tree is the source of the familiar sweet spicy smell used so sparingly in DELIGHT. This widely known spice adds force to the mixture and leaves a lingering, warm scent on the skin.

Pine balsam is the contrast scent that adds roundness to the composition. An ancient perfume, pine balsam has long been used to refresh and cleanse the skin; it gives DELIGHT a wonderful out-of-doors finish.

19

DELIGHT — fragrance of summer days and simple indulgences. Utterly charming.

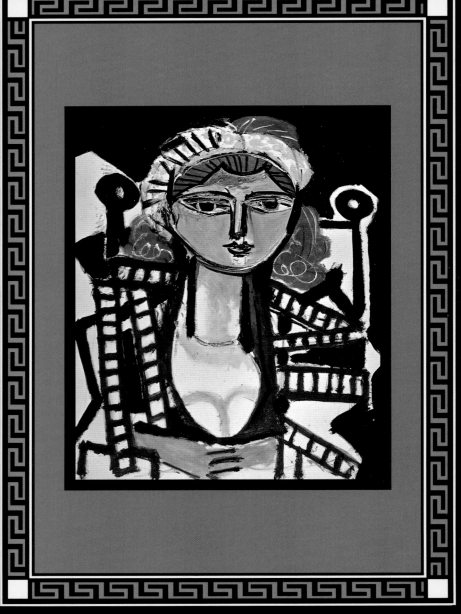

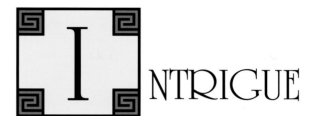

INTRIGUE

A potent and uninhibited

orchestration of rare aromas:

Musk, Ambergris, a whisper of

Frankincense, and a

penetrating top note of Jasmine.

A perfume that weaves an

intoxicating spell over all

who come near.

INTRIGUE, a distinctively sensual perfume, is a blend of provocative fragrances. Ambergris, long favored in perfumery for its superior fixative qualities, provides a soft yet spirited note that enhances a woman's natural scent. In turn, the aromas of frankincense, jasmine, and myrrh emerge very slowly to embrace the senses.

In the late 1970s, designer Sonia Rykiel, known for her stylish day-to-evening wear, created the equally attractive perfume, Seven Scents. In Seven Scents, the deep, sensual notes of musk and ambergris were blended with the top notes of ylang-ylang, gardenia, and tuberose to produce an arresting bouquet. INTRIGUE is a tribute to this versatile perfume.

> *40 Drops of Oil of Ambergris*
> *16 Drops of Oil of Jasmine*
> *8 Drops of Oil of Musk*
> *4 Drops of Oil of Frankincense*
> *Diluent to Fill a Quarter-Ounce Bottle*

Select a bottle for INTRIGUE that suggests artistry and sensuality. Perhaps you will discover a flask with golden threads of glass swirling upward over a base color of midnight blue or a flacon of geometrically cut crystal that perfectly fits the palm of your hand. The formula for INTRIGUE will yield one-quarter of an ounce.

Into a quarter-ounce bottle, drop the Oil of Ambergris, Oil of Jasmine, Oil of Musk, and Oil of Frankincense. Carefully pour or drop in the diluent to fill the bottle not quite to the top.

Seal the bottle and agitate it lightly to mix; transfer the mixture to your selected scent bottle with a perfumer's funnel. Age this perfume at least two days before dabbing it on, then anoint yourself with INTRIGUE before a chic party or enchanted evening for two. The feminine mystery of this scent will blend with your own to become irresistibly alluring.

The full, fascinating aroma of INTRIGUE comes from the sweet-scented oil of ambergris. One of perfumery's supreme fixatives, ambergris is the body note in INTRIGUE, where it combines perfectly with the mixture's complex woody, floral, and leather notes.

Jasmine provides a fragrant, beguiling note in perfume compositions, and has a vitalizing effect on the wearer. This unique and normally high floral note becomes subtle and sensuous in INTRIGUE.

Although known primarily as a fixative, musk can also be used as a single-note perfume. When used this way, it changes its scent according to the body chemistry of the wearer. Musk has a soft, sweet-leathery scent.

Frankincense, also known as olibanum, has a balsamic scent that is biting and aggressive, yet beckoning at the same time. Used in small doses in perfumes, this aromatic resin lends a soothing, woody note to the composition. It is also a familiar fragrance in incense.

23

INTRIGUE is the scent of mystery and romance — for the woman who loves to create a sensation.

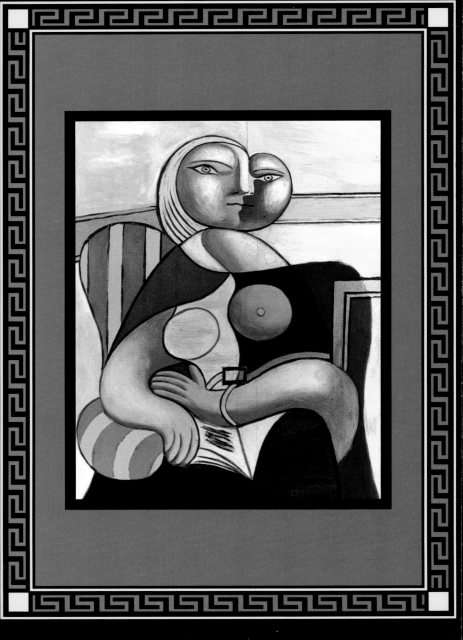

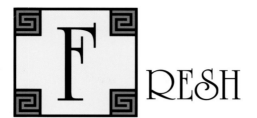

FRESH

A youthful and light composition

that enchants every day,

anywhere. Top notes of sunny

Lemongrass, sweet Orange

Blossom, and heavenly Rose are

held aloft by the

green and woody scents of

Rosemary and Sandalwood.

25

All the elements of a classic eau de cologne are celebrated in FRESH. Fine floral oils and a tart citrus essence are blended to create the impishly elusive scent of an early morning breeze.

The House of Guerlain is perhaps the oldest and most honored name in the perfume industry. One of its earliest fragrances, Eau de Cologne Imperiale, was created by Pierre-François-Pascal Guerlain for the Empress Eugénie in 1853. Like FRESH, this royal cologne combined orange blossom and lemon with rosemary to fashion a signature scent of timeless beauty.

24 Drops of Oil of Sandalwood
20 Drops of Oil of Orange Blossom
12 Drops of Oil of Rose
8 Drops of Oil of Cinnamon
4 Drops of Oil of Rosemary
4 Drops of Oil of Lemongrass
Diluent to Fill a One-Ounce Bottle

26

The original Eau de Cologne Imperiale was packaged in an elaborately wrought bottle with a bee, symbol of the industrious Napoleonic house, molded into it. Select a distinctive old-fashioned bottle, perhaps one on a pedestal with an aerosol bulb attached. FRESH is mixed as a toilet water and will yield one ounce.

Into a one-ounce bottle, drop the Oil of Sandalwood, Oil of Orange Blossom, Oil of Rose, Oil of Cinnamon, Oil of Rosemary, and Oil of Lemongrass. Carefully pour or drop in the

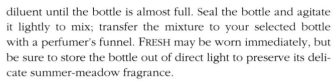

diluent until the bottle is almost full. Seal the bottle and agitate it lightly to mix; transfer the mixture to your selected bottle with a perfumer's funnel. FRESH may be worn immediately, but be sure to store the bottle out of direct light to preserve its delicate summer-meadow fragrance.

The woody warmth of sandalwood perfectly accompanies the light florals in FRESH. This fixative oil, extracted from the heartwood of the sandalwood tree, inspires an uplifting mood and adds a mysteriously sweet undertone to the blend.

The rich scent of rose is the embodiment of perfume itself and is the most widely used of all the essential oils. The fragrance is joyful, complex, and most decidedly feminine.

Orange blossom oil is collected from the large white blossom of the bitter orange tree, also known as the Seville orange. In perfumery, it is known as neroli oil, and its calming scent gracefully balances the exuberance of rose.

The oil derived from the bark of the cinnamon tree, also known as cassia oil, provides the spicy essence in FRESH. Its soft, sensual effect is subtle and warming, just like the caress of a spring breeze.

27

Rosemary has a keen piny note that makes it a wonderful component in colognes for both men and women. Its invigorating aroma brings a fine green note to FRESH.

Lemongrass, derived from a tropical grass, imparts a strong citrus snap to any fragrance. Lemongrass is brilliantly refreshing and, combined with rosemary, has a stimulating effect.

Splash on FRESH in the morning — and live the essence of youth all day long.

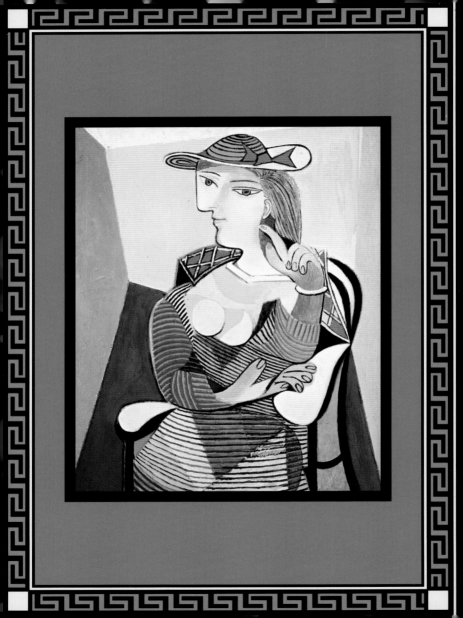

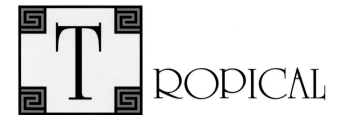

TROPICAL

Prepare for a heady

jungle-flower adventure.

The compelling scents of

Gardenia, Ylang-Ylang,

Frangipani, and a burst of

sweet Cassis float above the

earthy Patchouli and

Cedarwood base.

T ROPICAL is a rich and fascinating blend of exotic rain-
washed essences. Scents of ripened fruits and jungle flowers hover just above a deep woody note of cedar, suggesting
the luxury and relaxation of a color-rich tropical island.

The tropical fragrance, Amazone, was developed in the
1960s by the House of Hermès. Amazone was blended with a
cedar base to balance its volatile fruit and floral notes. The perfume was a sensation in France, where its intensity appealed to
the sybaritic and stylish Parisians. Like Amazone, TROPICAL is a
celebration of fine jungle essences.

> *30 Drops of Oil of Cassis*
> *20 Drops of Oil of Frangipani*
> *14 Drops of Oil of Patchouli*
> *12 Drops of Oil of Gardenia*
> *4 Drops of Oil of Ylang-ylang*
> *4 Drops of Oil of Cedarwood*
> *Diluent to Fill a Quarter-Ounce Bottle*

30

TROPICAL is mixed perfume strength and will yield one-quarter
of an ounce. Choose a small bottle that will reflect its rich floral
scent — perhaps a cut-crystal flacon that shows off its deep
amber color.

Into a quarter-ounce bottle, drop the Oil of Cassis, Oil of
Frangipani, Oil of Patchouli, Oil of Gardenia, Oil of Ylang-
ylang, and Oil of Cedarwood. Carefully pour or drop in the diluent until it nearly reaches the top of the bottle. Seal the bottle
and agitate it lightly to mix. With a perfumer's funnel, transfer it

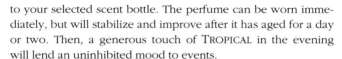

to your selected scent bottle. The perfume can be worn immediately, but will stabilize and improve after it has aged for a day or two. Then, a generous touch of TROPICAL in the evening will lend an uninhibited mood to events.

Cassis gives the high, exotic florals in TROPICAL a rounded, fruity base. Oil of cassis is extracted from the black currants of this European shrub. Its fruit is also used to make a popular sweet liqueur.

Frangipani is the name of the scent derived from the red jasmine. This essence has an interesting leathery note beneath its beautiful, sweet-and-spice fragrance.

Patchouli is used as a fixative in many of the world's most prized perfumes. Its aromatic, musty woodiness gracefully balances the sweetness of flowery essences and adds a wonderful complexity to perfumes.

Gardenia's scent rises slowly from the skin and imparts a most intoxicating afternote. A native flower of China, the gardenia's poignant scent is found in many Oriental blends.

Ylang-ylang has a sweet, almost bananalike aroma. Its scent is said to both uplift and relax the wearer. Growing in wild abundance throughout Indonesia, this cream-colored flower's essence is a mainstay of French perfumery.

The clean and fresh scent of cedarwood complements the patchouli, and gives the floral and fruit essences a sustaining woody base. Cedarwood also acts as a fix for the perfume, so that the higher notes retain their vibrancy.

Experience TROPICAL — an instant sensory getaway to a bright jungle paradise.

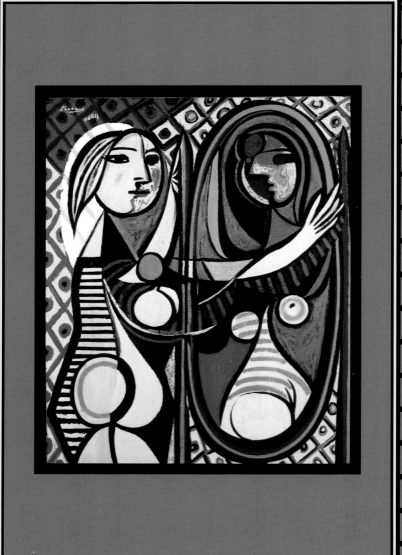

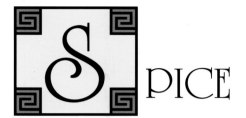 PICE

The romance of the Orient

captured in a fragrance:

East Indian Sandalwood,

West Indian Bergamot,

Patchouli from Southeast Asia,

made piquant with

Carnation.

A scent for the adventurous.

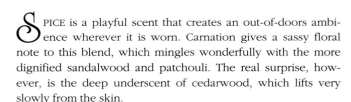

$\mathcal{S}$ PICE is a playful scent that creates an out-of-doors ambience wherever it is worn. Carnation gives a sassy floral note to this blend, which mingles wonderfully with the more dignified sandalwood and patchouli. The real surprise, however, is the deep underscent of cedarwood, which lifts very slowly from the skin.

Fragrances known as the spicy ambers first gained fame in 1928, when Sarah Bernhardt began to wear Soir de Paris. Soir de Paris was created by Alexandre Bourjois, who made the face powders and rouges favored by stage actresses of the time. The blend of carnation, sandalwood, and a chorus of light florals combined with mellow amber rapidly became the "in" fragrance among theatergoers along the Champs Elysées.

> *30 Drops of Oil of Bergamot*
> *18 Drops of Oil of Carnation*
> *18 Drops of Oil of Sandalwood*
> *12 Drops of Oil of Patchouli*
> *6 Drops of Oil of Cedarwood*
> *Diluent to Fill a Quarter-Ounce Bottle*

34

SPICE deserves a flask with personality. A small square- or oval-shaped bottle with a tightly fitted stopper is ideal. Thick, textured glass with a light tint of amber will preserve the strength of this scent while it accompanies you on your out-of-doors adventures. SPICE is mixed as a perfume and will yield one-quarter of an ounce.

Into a quarter-ounce bottle, drop the Oil of Bergamot, Oil

of Carnation, Oil of Sandalwood, Oil of Patchouli, and Oil of Cedarwood. Carefully pour or drop in the diluent until the bottle is nearly full. Seal the bottle and agitate it lightly to mix, then transfer it to your selected scent bottle with a perfumer's funnel. Age SPICE for at least two days. When it's ready to wear, you'll dazzle your admiring public with your vivacious aura.

Carnation owes its lively, spicy kick to eugenol, an element found in both clove and carnation oil. Because of this similarity in smell, carnation is also known as the "clove pink." It provides the bewitching top note in SPICE.

Bergamot is a fresh and stimulating fragrance. Its lovely scent is obtained from the skin of bergamot fruit, and its refreshing fruit-and-floral scent adds a sunny note of the outdoors to the composition.

The euphoric and embracing essence of sandalwood is the base note of many great perfumes. This sweet-smelling Oriental fragrance balances the blend and leaves a lingering, warm scent on the skin.

The thick dark oil of patchouli adds a stimulating and luxurious base scent to SPICE. The oil is extracted from the leaves of the patchouli tree from Southeast Asia.

Cedarwood oil is possibly the most ancient of the plant extracts. This balsamic oil has properties similar to those of sandalwood, but its scent is much less rounded. Cedarwood adds a clever low note to SPICE and is noticeable only at first, as the mist of scent rises from the skin.

SPICE is the scent of daring deeds — for the woman with worlds to conquer!

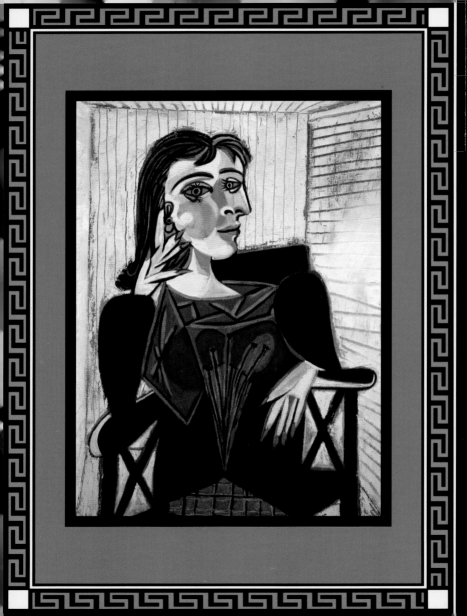

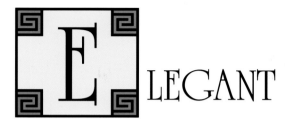

ELEGANT

A worldly perfume

with a hypnotic attraction.

The subtle essence of Oakmoss

is combined with fragrant

Bergamot and ethereal Amber

to create a scent that

lingers in the mind

long after it is gone.

E LEGANT is an enduring classic among perfumes. Its composition is known in perfumery as a chypre, named after the
island of Cypress, the mythical birthplace of Venus. Chypres
are a family of perfumes that have a soft, warm, honey-sweet
fragrance. Among the classic chypre essences in ELEGANT are
the heavenly scented base of oakmoss and the fresh citrus
brush of bergamot.

François Coty was the prolific originator of unique fragrances that later proved to be landmarks in the development
of perfumery. In 1917, Coty introduced to Parisian society a
scent he named Chypre. It became an immediate success, and
a new family of perfumes was born.

> *24 Drops of Oil of Oakmoss*
>
> *18 Drops of Oil of Bergamot*
>
> *12 Drops of Oil of Amber*
>
> *12 Drops of Oil of Vetiver*
>
> *6 Drops of Oil of Pine Balsam*
>
> *Diluent to Fill a Quarter-Ounce Bottle*

Coty took great pride in the presentation of his perfumes. He
linked his famous name with another well-known contemporary, René Lalique, whose Art Nouveau–style glassware was
decorated with motifs from nature — flowers, ferns, even Gre-
cian maidens. So depart from the usual, and select a small flask
with the refined grace and dazzling charm of the Belle Epoque.
ELEGANT is formulated as a perfume and will yield one-quarter
of an ounce.

Into a quarter-ounce bottle, drop the Oil of Oakmoss, Oil of Bergamot, Oil of Amber, Oil of Vetiver, and Oil of Pine Balsam. Carefully drop or pour in the diluent until the bottle is not quite full. Seal the bottle and agitate it lightly to mix; use a perfumer's funnel to transfer the liquid to your selected bottle. You will have to wait at least three days to wear this scent; the distinction of elegance requires restraint.

The powdery smell of oakmoss forms the base of ELEGANT. Its honeyed aroma releases slowly from the skin and gives ELEGANT a highly sought-after quality in a perfume — the ability to surround the wearer with a delicate mist of scent.

Bergamot's light, citrus snap is invariably the top note in any chypre perfume. This animated scent balances the aromatic composition and counters the hypnotic warmth of oakmoss and amber.

Amber has a round, dulcet tone that lends itself to so many perfumes. The resin this oil is processed from can be found in the bazaars of Morocco and Egypt. Amber resin releases its fragrance gracefully when rubbed against the warmth of the skin.

Vetiver's aroma is dry and earthy, yet it simultaneously suggests coolness. This complex fixative captures the scent of the sun-baked island of Cyprus in a single fragrance.

Pine balsam is reminiscent of the green, piny scent of sun-drenched cypress trees. The fragrance supports the high floral note of bergamot and adds roundness to the composition.

ELEGANT — an aromatic statement of balance and good taste. Rich. Boundless. Ethereal.

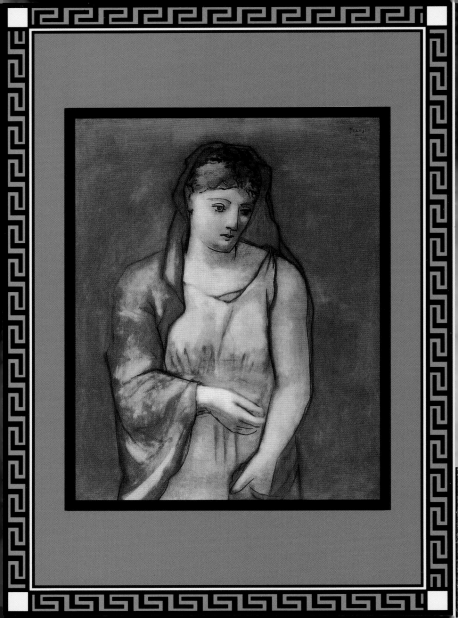

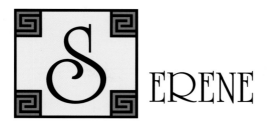

SERENE

A symphony of intoxicating

Rose ~ the fragrance

celebrated by the Sufi poets

of Persia ~ orchestrated

with Musk and a lilting

note of Sandalwood.

An intricate and elevating

enchantment.

$\mathcal{S}$ ERENE is an aromatic celebration of roses in every nuance of fragrance. The composition is a blend of three of the Near East's most precious scents — rose, musk, and sandalwood. The fresh green scent of rose geranium brings a resonant note of complexity to the perfume, which is further enhanced by the addition of sensuous musk and bewitching sandalwood.

Haute couturier Cristobal Balenciaga's genius for combining simplicity with luxury made him a legend in the world of fashion. He released his premier perfume, Le Dix, in 1947. This gorgeous rose-centered scent was actually a combination of soft florals — rose, jasmine, and iris — balanced by an earthy base of patchouli, sandalwood, and vetiver. SERENE was inspired by this classic perfume.

> *40 Drops of Oil of Rose*
> *30 Drops of Oil of Rose Geranium*
> *12 Drops of Oil of Sandalwood*
> *4 Drops of Oil of Musk*
> *Diluent to Fill a Quarter-Ounce Bottle*

SERENE is composed as a perfume and will yield one-quarter of an ounce. The perfume is nearly colorless and is beautiful when contained in a translucent bottle. The purity of a porcelain or milk-glass flacon is also ideal for SERENE. Perhaps you will even find one with a hand-painted rose adorning it.

Into a quarter-ounce bottle, drop the Oil of Rose, Oil of

Rose Geranium, Oil of Sandalwood, and Oil of Musk. Carefully pour or drop in the diluent until it nearly reaches the top. Seal the bottle and agitate it lightly to mix. With a perfumer's funnel, transfer the mixture to your selected bottle. SERENE will be too "green" to wear immediately, and must age for two days. Then, dab it on and disarm those around you with the simple — yet luxurious — scent of SERENE.

The unmistakable fragrance of rose has long been used to enhance femininity. The oil of this "queen of flowers" has a cool, green aroma, which is soothing and uplifting to the spirit.

The scented geranium produces many different fragrances — rose geranium is one of the most popular. This lively rose scent is both earthy and stimulating, adding a refreshing and harmonious note to the blend.

The oil of the sandalwood tree is highly valued as a fixative and as a perfume in its own right. Mysore sandalwood oil of East India is considered the very best, and the trees that produce it are prized and protected by the government of India.

Heady and seductive oil of musk is one of the most sought-after fixatives in the world of perfumery. It lends an opulent base note to any perfume and responds to the mood of the individual who wears it.

Bask in SERENE by day or by night — for the woman who creates the mood of the moment.

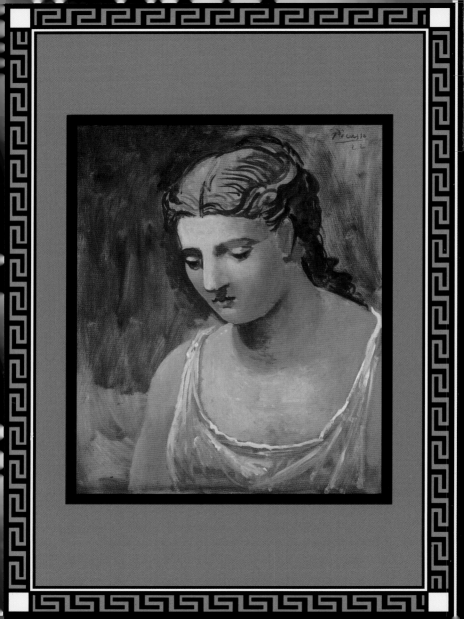

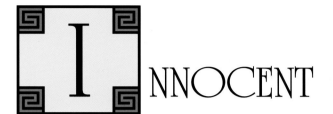

INNOCENT

A tender flower poem, this

disarming concoction is destined

to enchant far and wide.

Celebrate a Victorian bouquet

of timeless floral notes: Lilac,

Heliotrope, and Violet.

Deliciously subtle, utterly

beguiling.

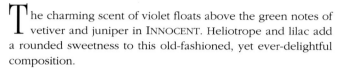

The charming scent of violet floats above the green notes of vetiver and juniper in INNOCENT. Heliotrope and lilac add a rounded sweetness to this old-fashioned, yet ever-delightful composition.

In 1892, Roger et Gallet, one of the oldest perfume manufacturers in France, introduced a beautiful perfume called Vera Violetta. Parma violets, meticulously picked by hand, were used in the formula. To this day, violets are cultivated for this purpose and their essences are distilled at the Parma monastery of San Giovanni Evangelista in Italy. INNOCENT was formulated to evoke the fine violet waters favored by the fashionable women of long ago.

> *40 Drops of Oil of Violet*
> *12 Drops of Oil of Heliotrope*
> *8 Drops of Oil of Vetiver*
> *4 Drops of Oil of Juniper*
> *4 Drops of Oil of Lilac*
> *Diluent to Fill a Quarter-Ounce Bottle*

INNOCENT is a very delicate perfume that must be protected from the light. Choose a small dark blue or amber or ruby-glass bottle — perhaps one with an etched floral motif. A flask of Victorian design would be an ideal package for this precious fragrance. INNOCENT is formulated as a perfume and will yield one-quarter of an ounce.

Into a quarter-ounce bottle, drop the Oil of Violet, Oil of Heliotrope, Oil of Vetiver, Oil of Juniper, and Oil of Lilac. Carefully pour or drop in the diluent, filling the bottle almost to the top. Seal the bottle and agitate it lightly to mix, then transfer the perfume to your selected bottle with a perfumer's funnel. INNOCENT requires a day of aging to round out the high floral notes into a full-blossomed nosegay.

The essential oil of violet is extracted from *Viola odorata*, or the Parma violet. Its disarming scent has been a treasured fragrance since the seventeenth century and is included in many floral perfumes.

Heliotrope's exquisitely mellow floral note complements the fragile essence of violet. The word *heliotrope* means "to turn toward the sun," which describes a characteristic of this fragrant South American flower.

Vetiver oil is extracted from the roots of a tropical Asian grass. The fragrances in floral blends become elevated with the addition of vetiver. With its dry, peppery scent, vetiver enhances the high notes in floral blends, elevating them to the angelic.

Juniper acts as a fixative and gives the composition a green, slightly piny zest. Extracted from the berries produced by the shrub, juniper oil has a calming effect on the wearer.

47

In Victorian England, the scent of lilacs symbolized new love. This beautiful climbing shrub is traditionally planted at the rear of English herb gardens to capture the natural perfumes growing there.

Touch on INNOCENT and surround yourself with the aura and beauty of a romantic garden.

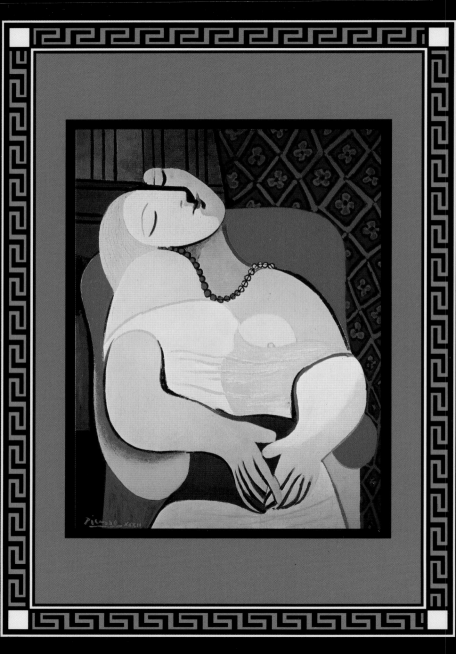

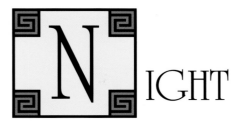

NIGHT

This penetrating, special-occasion scent features Jasmine, the precious flower that exudes its most intense perfume just before dawn. The alluring bouquet is rounded with Amber and Vanilla, and underscored by a woody note of Patchouli. Unforgettable.

N IGHT is a deep, rich, and intriguing formula known to perfumers as an Oriental blend. The aroma surrounds you
with the black velvet beauty of evening. A golden, sweet note
of amber rounds the fragrance and brings true elegance to the
composition.

The House of Guerlain presented the archetype of the
modern Oriental blend, Shalimar, in 1925. Jacques Guerlain,
the master himself, created this sumptuous blend. A beloved
classic, it is treasured among perfume lovers the world over.
Dana followed Guerlain's lead with Tabu, another Oriental fragrance that remains popular today.

> *18 Drops of Oil of Patchouli*
> *9 Drops of Oil of Vanilla*
> *9 Drops of Oil of Amber*
> *30 Drops of Oil of Orange Blossom*
> *18 Drops of Oil of Jasmine*
> *Diluent to Fill a Quarter-Ounce Bottle*

NIGHT is composed as a perfume and will yield one-quarter of
an ounce. Choose a small bottle, perhaps a flacon of hard,
black glass. You may find a shape reminiscent of the East, such
as a lotus bud or a pagoda that will display the scent in the
imaginative way that it deserves.

Into a quarter-ounce bottle, drop the Oil of Patchouli, Oil
of Vanilla, Oil of Amber, Oil of Orange Blossom, and Oil of Jasmine. Carefully pour or drop in the diluent until it almost
reaches the top. Seal the bottle and agitate it lightly to mix;

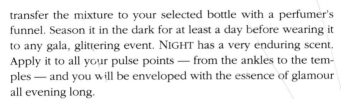

transfer the mixture to your selected bottle with a perfumer's funnel. Season it in the dark for at least a day before wearing it to any gala, glittering event. NIGHT has a very enduring scent. Apply it to all your pulse points — from the ankles to the temples — and you will be enveloped with the essence of glamour all evening long.

Precious oil of jasmine, originally transported out of Persia and the high mountain ranges of India's Kashmir region, is now grown commercially in France and in other temperate areas. All of the European *grands parfums* include jasmine in their formulas.

Patchouli possesses an extremely rich, spicy odor. It is a haunting scent but, like vetiver, it is not a pretty one in and of itself. Patchouli is an important ingredient in all Oriental blends, and is well known as a fixative.

Amber is actually a blend of oils from several tree resins, skillfully mixed to emit a complex, but subtle, sweet odor. It is often worn as a single-note perfume, but when blended with other fragrances it acts to center and mellow the composition.

Orange blossom has a delicate airiness that is far more flowery than the simple citrus note of the peel. It is an extraordinarily elegant scent, widely used in eau de cologne. The scent of orange blossom is soothing, refreshing, and uplifting.

51

The vanilla plant is a climbing orchid, native to Mexico. Vanilla adds sweetness and depth to the composition. The scent has great tenacity, lingering on the skin for a very long time.

NIGHT comes alive in the evening — wear it to shine in the dark.

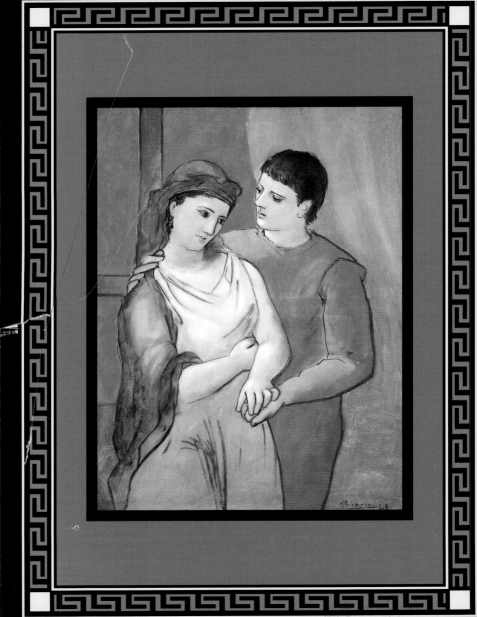

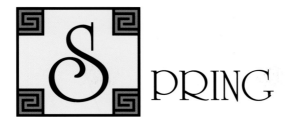

SPRING

An outdoor note of
Lavender is combined
with the clean scent of
Rosemary and topped with
the gloriously fragrant
Tuberose.
Bright and fresh,
invigorating and inviting.

$\mathcal{S}$ PRING is a joyfully fresh fragrance that is known among perfumers as a "green scent." The beautiful floral note of tuberose in this formula calls to mind the first blossom of the season.

In 1917, François Coty created the perfume sensation L'Origan, as a tribute to Coco Chanel and her impact on the women's fashion of the time — a fragrance that reflected the smart, well-bred look of the British aristocracy that she so admired. The genius of this fragrance is recaptured in SPRING.

> *30 Drops of Oil of Lavender*
> *8 Drops of Oil of Rosemary*
> *20 Drops of Oil of Tuberose*
> *16 Drops of Oil of Oakmoss*
> *Diluent to Fill a One-Ounce Bottle*

Select a perfume bottle that suggests to you the lighthearted feeling of early spring. Because this fragrance is mixed as a toilet water rather than a full-strength perfume, you may wish to use a bottle with an aerosol bulb attached so you can spray the air around you and allow the fragrance to cling all over. The formula for SPRING will yield one ounce.

54

Into a one-ounce bottle, drop the Oil of Lavender, Oil of Rosemary, Oil of Tuberose, and Oil of Oakmoss. Carefully pour or drop in the diluent to fill the bottle not quite to the top. Seal the bottle and agitate it lightly to mix; decant it into your decorative scent bottle with a perfumer's funnel. Put the perfume aside, out of direct light, and allow it to season over-night. Tomorrow, you'll want to experience this scent first thing in the morning. The effect? Green as a crushed leaf and ever so delicately floral.

European perfumery has made great use of lavender's fresh outdoor note in colognes and sachets. Lavender's scent is refreshingly herbal with a decided floral undertone and a calming, balancing effect.

Rosemary provides a sportive, clean scent and has a stimulating effect that complements lavender's calming one. Rosemary is one of the most important of the herbal oils used in the manufacture of perfume.

Long after it is applied, the scent of tuberose will hover over your skin. A native of Mexico, the white blossoms of this plant were known to the Aztec apothecaries as "bone flower." The odor of tuberose is intensely sweet, but with an exotic camphorlike note.

Finally, oakmoss, which is a resin of lichen, has a scent reminiscent of freshly cut hay with a rich, honeyed undertone. Oakmoss acts as a fixative to maintain the integrity of each of the individual oils and allows the perfume to work in harmony with your body heat, releasing the scent as a single combined fragrance.

55

Enjoy SPRING as a daytime splash — ideal for the active woman. Perfect for both work and play.

YOUR OWN FRAGRANCE FORMULA

....
....
....
....
....
....
....
....
....
....
....
....
....
....
....
....

YOUR OWN FRAGRANCE FORMULA

....

....

....

....

....

....

....

....

....

....

....

....

....

....

....

....

....

YOUR OWN FRAGRANCE FORMULA

....

....

....

....

....

....

....

....

....

....

....

....

....

....

....

....

....

Essential Oils Shopping Guide

Stores marked with an asterisk have outlets
at a number of locations.

Aroma Therapy Products
P.O. Box 2354
Fair Oaks, CA 95628
(916) 965-7546

Aroma Vera
2728 South Robertson Boulevard
Los Angeles, CA 90034
(213) 280-0407

* Aveda
509 Madison Avenue
New York, NY 10022
(212) 832-2416

John Bell & Croyden
Department A6 Mo
52-54 Wigmore Street
London W.I., England
44-71-935-5555

Belle Star, Inc.
23151 Alcalde, #C4
Laguna Hills, CA 92653
800-442-7827

* The Body Shop
1341 Seventh Street
Berkeley, CA 94710
(415) 524-0360

* The Body Shop International Ltd
Hawthorn Road
Little Hampton, West Sussex BN17 7LR, England
44-0903-726-250

The Body Shop by Mail
45 Horsehill Road
Cedar Knolls, NJ 07927
800-541-2535

* Caswell-Massey Company
111 Eighth Avenue
New York, NY 10011
800-326-0500

Cherchez
862 Lexington Avenue
New York, NY 10021
(212) 737-8313

Common Scents
39020 A 24th Street
San Francisco, CA 94114
(415) 826-1019

Culpeper Ltd
21 Bruton Street
London W1X 7DA, England
44-71-499-2406

Czech & Speake
39c Jermyn Street
London SW1 6JH, England
44-71-439-0216

The Essential Oil Co.
P.O. Box 88
Sandy, OR 97055
(503) 695-2400

Farmaceutica de Santa Maria Novella
Via della Scala, 16
50123, Florence, Italy

Floris
89 Jerymn Street
London SW1 6JH, England
44-71-930-2885

Floris
703 Madison Avenue
New York, NY 10021
(212) 935-9100

Green Mountain Herbs Ltd
P.O. Box 2369
Boulder, CO 80306
800-525-2696

Hove Parfumeur
723 Toulouse Street
New Orleans, LA 70130
(504) 525-7827

Kiehl's Pharmacy
109 Third Avenue
New York, NY 10003
(212) 475-3400

Madini Oils
68F Tinker Street
Woodstock, NY 12498
(914) 679-7647

Original Swiss Aromatics
P.O. Box 606
San Rafael, CA 94915
(415) 459-3998

Palmetto
1034 Montana Avenue
Santa Monica, CA 90403
(213) 395-6687

Ra-Bob International
320 Hillsdale Drive
Wichita, KS 67230
(316) 733-0904

Uncommon Scents, Inc.
555 High Street
Eugene, OR 97401
(503) 345-0952

Grateful acknowledgment is made for permission to
reproduce the following paintings
by Pablo Picasso:

Page 16: *Woman with a Book,* 1932, The Norton
Simon Foundation.

Page 20: *Woman in a Green Dress,* 1954, Spadem
/Art Resource, New York.

Page 24: *La Lecture,* 1932, Musée Picasso, Paris,
Spadem/Art Resource, New York.

Page 28: *Seated Woman,* 1937, Private Collection,
Scala/Art Resource, New York.

Page 32: *Girl Before a Mirror,* 1932, The Museum of
Modern Art, New York.

Page 36: *Portrait of Dora Maar,* Musée Picasso,
Paris, Giraudon/Art Resource, New York.

Page 40: *Woman with a Blue Veil,* Los Angeles
County Museum of Art.

Page 44: *Classical Head,* 1922, National Gallery of
Art, Washington, D.C.

Page 48: *The Dream,* 1932, V. W. Ganz, Giraudon
/Art Resource, New York.

Page 52: *The Lovers,* 1923, National Gallery of Art,
Washington, D.C.